About the NCCN Guidelines for Patients®

NCCN National Comprehensive Cancer Network®

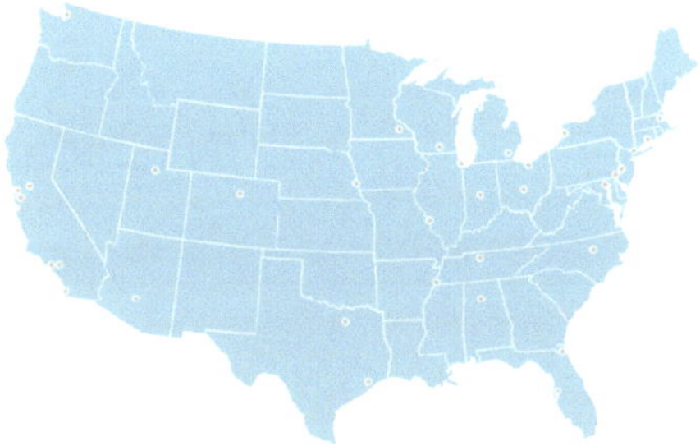

Did you know that top cancer centers across the United States work together to improve cancer care? This alliance of leading cancer centers is called the National Comprehensive Cancer Network® (NCCN®).

Cancer care is always changing. NCCN develops evidence-based cancer care recommendations used by health care providers worldwide. These frequently updated recommendations are the NCCN Clinical Practice Guidelines in Oncology (NCCN Guidelines®). The NCCN Guidelines for Patients plainly explain these expert recommendations for people with cancer and caregivers.

These NCCN Guidelines for Patients are based on the NCCN Clinical Practice Guidelines in Oncology (NCCN Guidelines®) for Small Cell Lung Cancer, Version 3.2024 — June 11, 2024.

View the NCCN Guidelines for Patients free online
NCCN.org/patientguidelines

Find an NCCN Cancer Center near you
NCCN.org/cancercenters

Connect with us

Supporters

NATIONAL COMPREHENSIVE CANCER NETWORK®
NCCN FOUNDATION
Guiding Treatment. Changing Lives.

NCCN Guidelines for Patients are supported by funding from the NCCN Foundation®

NCCN Foundation gratefully acknowledges the following corporate supporters for helping to make available these NCCN Guidelines for Patients: AstraZeneca.

NCCN independently adapts, updates, and hosts the NCCN Guidelines for Patients. Our corporate supporters do not participate in the development of the NCCN Guidelines for Patients and are not responsible for the content and recommendations contained therein.

To make a gift or learn more, visit online or email

NCCNFoundation.org/donate

PatientGuidelines@NCCN.org

Contents

NCCN Foundation seeks to support the millions of patients and their families affected by a cancer diagnosis by funding and distributing NCCN Guidelines for Patients. NCCN Foundation is also committed to advancing cancer treatment by funding the nation's promising doctors at the center of innovation in cancer research. For more details and the full library of patient and caregiver resources, visit NCCN.org/patients.

National Comprehensive Cancer Network (NCCN) and NCCN Foundation
3025 Chemical Road, Suite 100, Plymouth Meeting, PA 19462 USA

1
Lung cancer basics

Small cell lung cancer forms from cells that line the inner airways of the lungs. It's a cancer that can be aggressive and grows fast. This chapter gives you the basics of small cell lung cancer.

What is lung cancer?

The lungs are the main organs of the respiratory system. They deliver oxygen to the blood and remove carbon dioxide from the blood. The transfer of these gases in and out of the body is called respiration.

Lung cancers form from cells that line the airways of the lungs. The lungs' airways are called the bronchus, bronchioli, and alveoli.

Cancer cells don't behave like normal cells. They break the rules of cell growth.

- Cancer cells make many new cancer cells. They also do not die when they should. This overgrowth of cancer cells becomes a mass of tissue called a tumor.
- Cancer cells grow out of control. They can grow through the airway and into the lung tissue. They can grow through the lung wall and invade other body parts.
- Cancer cells can break away from a tumor and spread. They can enter the bloodstream or a fluid called lymph and spread to other places.

This out-of-control cell growth can harm the body. Cancer cells crowd out and overwhelm normal cells. Without enough normal cells, cancer cells can cause organs to stop working.

Scientists have learned a great deal about cancer. As a result, today's treatments work

Small cell lung cancer cells appear small and blue when viewed with a microscope.

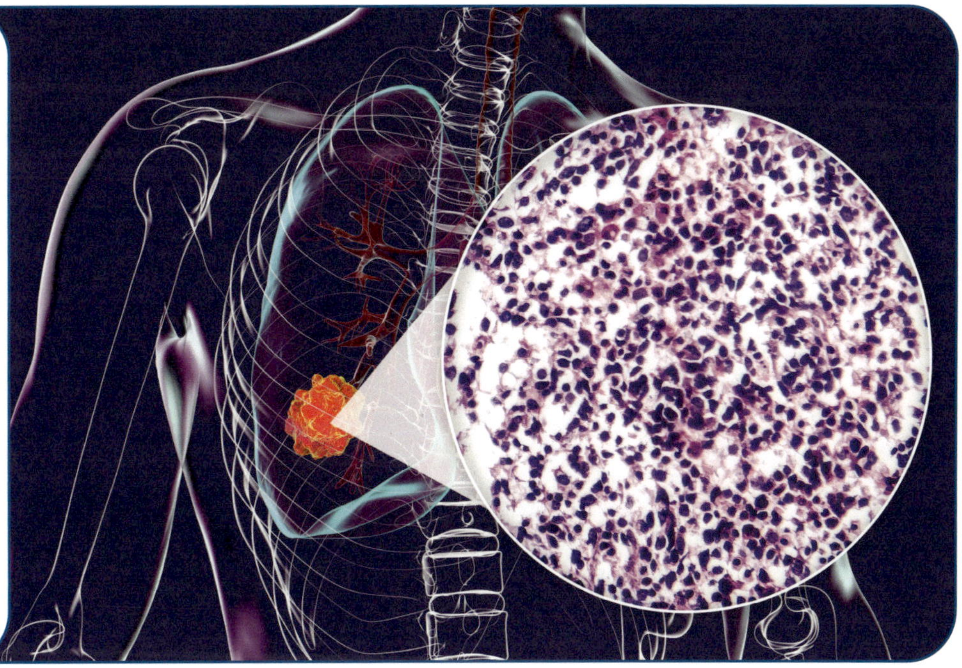

better than treatments in the past. Also, many people with cancer have more than one treatment option.

The two most common types of lung cancer are:

- Non-small cell lung cancer (NSCLC), further divided into:
  - Adenocarcinoma
  - Squamous cell carcinoma
  - Adenosquamous carcinoma
  - Large cell carcinoma
  - Sarcomatoid carcinoma
- Small cell lung cancer (SCLC), further divided into:
  - Small cell carcinoma
  - Combined (small and non-small) cell lung carcinoma

The names of the cancers refer to their appearance under a microscope. When viewed with a microscope, SCLCs appear small and blue.

Sometimes lung tumors contain both small cell and non-small cell lung cancer cells. These are called combined (small and non-small) cell lung carcinomas and are usually treated like small cell lung cancer.

SCLC is much less common than NSCLC. It is the focus of this book.

NCCN has a two-part book series on NSCLC, found at NCCN.org/patientguidelines and on the NCCN Patient Guides for Cancer app.

What are the causes and risk factors?

Smoking cigarettes is the main cause of SCLC. Almost everyone with SCLC smokes or has smoked. Many people with SCLC have regularly smoked more than a pack a day.

Exposure to second-hand smoke also increases the risk of lung cancer. Second-hand smoke is the smoke exhaled by another person and the smoke from combustible tobacco products.

Although rare in Western countries, there are occasions where people with no smoking history develop this disease.

There are other unknown causes of SCLC. Researchers are still learning why some people who smoke never get lung cancer and others who have never smoked do. A person's chances of getting SCLC are higher in the following situations:

- Over 70 years of age
- Prior radiation therapy to the chest
- Exposure to cancer-causing chemicals (also known as carcinogens), such as radon and asbestos

If you don't smoke, don't start. If you do smoke, quit. New lung tumors are less likely to develop after quitting smoking.

Nicotine addiction is one of the hardest addictions to stop. The stress of having cancer may make it even harder to quit. There is help. Ask your health care providers about counseling and medicines to help you quit.

What are the symptoms of SCLC?

SCLC can cause many types of symptoms. The symptoms depend on where the lung tumor has grown to or spread. SCLC can prevent the lungs from getting the air they need. Some people also have symptoms from paraneoplastic syndromes, which are caused by an abnormal body response to lung cancer.

Some symptoms caused by SCLC are listed in **Guide 1.**

SCLC is often found when it's causing symptoms or routine blood tests are abnormal.

Less often, it's found in x-rays or CT scans before symptoms start. Unlike other lung cancers, it's difficult to detect SCLC early because it grows more quickly.

Airways of the lungs

Air moves through your body in a series of airways. It travels down your throat and through the windpipe (trachea). The windpipe splits into 2 airways called bronchi. Inside the lung, each bronchus branches off into the parts of the lung, called lobes. The right lung has 3 lobes, and the left lung has 2 lobes. The bronchi divide into smaller airways called the bronchioli. At the end of the bronchioli are sacs called alveoli. Oxygen is transferred from air into the blood in the alveoli.

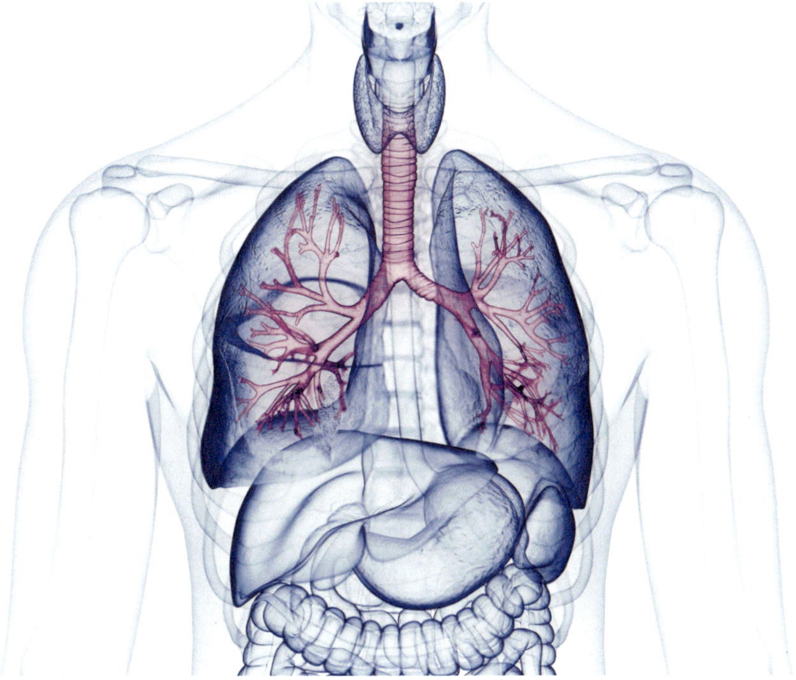

Your primary care provider may be the first to suspect that you have lung cancer. You will need to see specialists to determine if you have cancer. Your assessment team may include the following board-certified experts:

- Thoracic radiologist
- Interventional radiologist
- Pulmonologist
- Thoracic surgeon
- Medical oncologist
- Radiation oncologist

To confirm that you have cancer, you'll need testing of your body tissue or fluid. Small samples will be removed from your body during a procedure called a biopsy.

Guide 1
Symptoms of small cell lung cancer

Symptoms caused by the lung tumor	• Chronic cough • Bloody lung mucus • Wheezing
Symptoms caused by cancer spread in the chest	• Hoarse voice • Trouble swallowing • Chest pain • Swelling • Spinal pain • Enlarged chest veins • Trouble breathing • Feeling lightheaded • Lumps near the collarbone
Symptoms caused by cancer spread to the head	• Headache • Confusion • Slurred speech • Trouble walking • Lack of coordination • Weakness of a limb
Symptoms caused by cancer spread to the abdomen	• Pain • Yellow-colored eyes or skin • Fatigue • Burning or prickling feeling • Fever • Muscle weakness • Loss of bowel and bladder control

There are many types of biopsies for lung cancer. Some involve a needle while others require cutting through body tissue. Most biopsies are low-risk procedures and do not cause any long lasting harm.

Your health care providers will decide what biopsy is right for you and how they will test the removed tissue.

Getting a biopsy does not pose a risk for the cancer spreading.

What's the treatment for SCLC?

The best treatment for SCLC depends on the stage of the tumor, your health, and what medicines your body responds to. Further chapters describe treatment in detail.

Key points

- Cancer cells don't follow the rules of cell growth. They make many new cancer cells, invade nearby tissue, and spread to other body parts.
- The lungs help the body get the air it needs to live.
- Lung cancer often starts in the cells that line the airways.
- Small cell lung cancer (SCLC) grows fast and it has commonly spread outside the lung by the time it's found.
- Smoking cigarettes is the main cause of SCLC, but there are other unknown causes.
- Ask your health care provider for help to quit smoking. Quitting may improve treatment results and reduce side effects of treatment.
- SCLC is most often found when it's causing symptoms. Its symptoms depend on where the cancer is growing in the body.

2

Lung cancer staging

A cancer stage is a rating of the extent of cancer in the body. There are two staging systems for small-cell lung cancer. A combined system is better for treatment planning. This chapter describes these systems.

What is cancer staging?

At diagnosis, the degree of lung cancer growth and its spread differ between people. Cancer doctors needed a way to measure and compare different cancer tumors.

A staging system is a standard way of grouping lung cancers by their growth and spread. Health care providers use cancer staging to:

- Assess the possible outcome of the cancer, called the prognosis
- Identify and plan the best treatment options for you
- Study and compare different groups of cancer in research

> **“Cancer care involves a team effort among the various health care providers and the patient. It is essential to be knowledgeable about the cancer in order to make educated decisions regarding the care and treatment to be given. With so much on the Internet, much of which may be outdated, publications, such as this book, are essential to patients receiving accurate and timely information so that they further understand their disease and treatments."**

Lung cancer staging is based on the growth and spread of cancer cells. Lung cancer cells may:

- Form one or more tumors in the lung
- Grow through the lung wall and into other body tissue
- Spread to and form tumors in other organs

There are 2 staging systems for small cell lung cancer (SCLC).

- VA (Veterans Administration) system
- TNM (tumor, node, metastasis) system

What is the VA staging system?

The VA Lung Study Group created the first staging system for SCLC. It has been used in studies on treatment. The system divides lung cancer into 2 stages:

- Limited stage
- Extensive stage

Limited-stage cancer is found on one side of the chest and can be treated with radiation therapy. The cancer is contained in an area that would fit within one radiation field.

With modern radiation treatment techniques, the definition of limited-stage disease has been expanded to include some cases that are on both sides of the chest as long as they can be safely treated with radiation.

Most people with SCLC have extensive stage. Extensive-stage cancer can't be treated within one radiation field with the intent to cure the cancer. It has spread too much.

For example, it may have spread to the other side of the chest, to the fluid around the lungs or heart, or outside the chest.

What is the TNM staging system?

The TNM stages of SCLC range from stage 0 to stage 4. The more serious the cancer growth and spread, the higher the stage. Stage 0 cancers are only in the airways and are very rare.

Stage 1

Stage 1 cancers consist of one small lung tumor and have not spread to other body parts. Stage 1A tumors are 3 centimeters (cm, a little over 1 inch, or the size of a grape) or smaller. Stage 1B tumors are larger but don't exceed 4 cm (roughly an inch and a half, or the size of a walnut).

Stage 2

Stage 2A cancers are like stage 1 cancers except larger (up to 5 cm, just about 2 inches, the size of a lime). Stage 2B cancers are larger (up to 7 cm, about 2.75 inches, the size of a peach), have started to invade other body parts, or have multiple tumors in one lobe. Other 2B cancers consist of one lung tumor that is no larger than 5 cm and has spread to lymph nodes inside the lung.

Stage 3

Stage 3 is a mixed group of locally advanced cancers. They are further grouped as stages 3A, 3B, or 3C. Many of these cancers include:

- A large lung tumor that is 7 cm or larger
- A lung tumor that has markedly invaded other tissue
- Lung tumors in multiple lobes of the lung

- Cancer spread to lymph nodes between the lungs, in the other lung, or near the collarbone

Stage 4

The cancer has spread far from the main tumor. Stage 4A cancer has spread far within the chest or to only one place outside the chest. Stage 4B cancer has spread to at least two places outside the chest.

How does NCCN stage SCLC?

Most research studies on lung cancer treatment have used the VA system. The benefit of the TNM system is that it better identifies when local therapy—surgery or radiation—can be safely used. NCCN lung cancer experts use a combined staging approach to account for these factors.

- Limited stage includes cancers that are stages 1 to 3 and can be treated with radiation and chemotherapy.
- Extensive stage includes any cancers, including stage 4, that can't be treated with high radiation doses intended to cure.

Until the TNM system is more widely used in research studies, the best approach is a combined staging system. Cancer staging in the following chapters refers to this combined system.

Key points

- A cancer staging system is a standard way of grouping cancers by their growth and spread. Staging the cancer is needed before treatment.
- The VA (Veterans Administration) staging system groups cancers into either limited stage or extensive stage. It has been used the most in research studies on treatment of lung cancer.
- The TNM (tumor, node, metastasis) system groups cancers into stage 0, 1, 2, 3, or 4. This system allows for more precise treatment planning.
- NCCN experts of small cell lung cancer (SCLC) use a combined staging approach. Limited-stage cancers include stages 1 to 3, which can be treated with radiation therapy. Extensive-stage cancers, such as stage 4, can't be treated with high radiation doses intended to cure.

3
Tests for lung cancer

Your health care providers will order several tests to plan your treatment. Some tests assess your general health. Other tests assess the cancer. This chapter explains the tests in detail.

Health history and exams

Your cancer care providers need to have all your health information. One of the first steps is obtaining a complete report of your health called a medical history. Read **Guide 2** on page 16 for a full list of tests that are used to plan treatment.

Medical history

Your health care providers will ask about any health problems and treatments you've had. When you meet with your cancer health care providers, be ready to talk about:

- Illnesses
- Injuries
- Health conditions
- Symptoms
- Medications

Bring a list of old and new medications and any over-the-counter medicines, herbals, or supplements you take.

Be prepared to discuss the health problems of your close blood relatives. Such family members include siblings, parents, and grandparents. Although small cell lung cancer (SCLC) doesn't run in families, other cancers and health conditions can be hereditary. Your health care providers need to know about them.

Physical exam

After taking your health history, your health care provider will perform a physical exam. An exam is done to find signs of disease and decide which treatments may be options. During this exam, expect the following to be checked:

- Your body temperature
- Your blood pressure
- Your pulse and breathing rate
- Your weight
- How your lungs, heart, and gut sound
- How your eyes, skin, nose, ears, and mouth look
- Level of pain when you are touched

Performance status

Your health care providers will assess how well you can do day-to-day activities—like working, walking, or taking a shower. Your ability to do these activities is called a performance status.

The more activities you can do, the better your performance status. Your health care providers will use your performance status to assess if you can undergo certain treatments.

Performance status is often measured on a scale that ranges from 0 to 5. Lower scores mean better performance status.

Guide 2
Tests for small cell lung cancer

Health history and exams	• Medical history • Physical exam • Performance status
Blood tests	• Complete blood count (CBC) • Electrolytes • Liver function tests • Kidney function tests
Imaging	• Diagnostic CT of the chest, abdomen, and pelvis • MRI (preferred) or CT of the brain • PET/CT may be ordered by your health care provider • Bone imaging if needed
Staging biopsies	**If imaging suggests the cancer is limited stage, you may receive:** • Thoracentesis if there is pleural effusion • Thoracoscopy if thoracentesis results are unclear • Bone marrow biopsy and aspiration if blood work suggests cancer spread to bone marrow • Biopsy of mediastinal lymph nodes for limited stages 1 and 2A that will be treated with surgery or radiation therapy
Cancer cell tests	• Pathology review • Biomarker testing
Pulmonary function tests	• Spirometry • Gas diffusion test • Body plethysmograph

Blood tests

Blood tests measure blood cells, proteins, and chemicals in the bloodstream. Your health care providers will use these tests to assess your general health and if the cancer may have spread. They will plan other tests and cancer treatment based on test results.

A blood draw removes a sample of blood for testing. It is done with a needle inserted into a vein. The following tests are needed:

- A complete blood count (CBC) measures parts of the blood, including counts of white blood cells, red blood cells, and platelets.
- Electrolytes are minerals in the blood. They include sodium, calcium, and potassium. Organs, such as your bones, need electrolytes to work well.
- Liver function tests measure chemicals made or processed by the liver.
- Blood urea nitrogen (BUN) is waste made by your body after you eat. Too much BUN in blood could be a sign of kidney damage.
- Creatinine is waste made by muscles. Too much creatinine in blood could be a sign of kidney damage.

"Ask as many questions as possible and bring a family member with you to appointments."

Pulmonary function tests

To receive some treatments, your lungs have to work fairly well. Pulmonary function tests show how well lungs work.

- Spirometry involves blowing into a tube to measure how much air you breathe and how fast you breathe.
- A gas diffusion test involves breathing in a harmless gas and measuring how much you breathe out. It tells how much oxygen travels from your lungs into your blood.

Imaging

Imaging makes pictures of the insides of your body. It can show cancer in deep tissue, lymph nodes, or distant body parts outside of the lung. Imaging is helpful for cancer staging and treatment planning.

An injection of a contrast agent is sometimes used to make the pictures clearer. Contrast should not be used if you may be allergic to it. During imaging, you'll lie on a table that slides into the scanning machine. At least part of your body will be in the machine.

A radiologist is a health care provider who's an expert in reading images. They'll convey the test results to your care team.

CT of chest, abdomen, and pelvis

Most people first get a diagnostic CT of their chest, abdomen, and sometimes pelvis. This scan takes many pictures of your body from

Imaging

Imaging is used to make painless pictures of the insides of your body. You will lie on a table that will move into the tunnel of the machine. You will need to lie still during the scan. You may be asked to hold your breath. The scan is quick. The pictures will be viewed on a computer by a doctor who will look for signs of cancer.

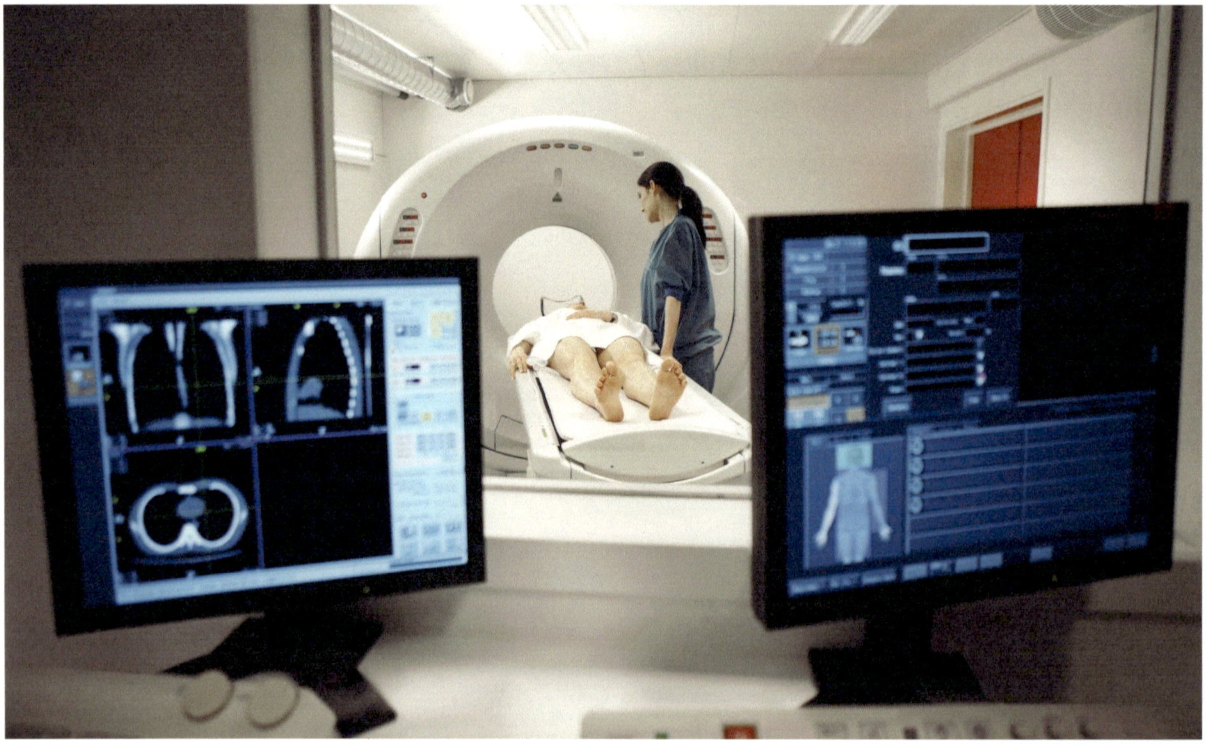

different angles using x-rays. Contrast will be used. A computer combines the pictures to make a 3D image.

Brain imaging

MRI can detect small tumors in the brain. It uses a magnetic field and radio waves to make pictures. Contrast will be used. If MRI can't be done, you may get a CT with contrast of your head.

PET/CT from skull base to knees

PET scans use a special camera that detects an injected radioactive sugar. Cancer cells quickly use the sugar. Combining PET with CT may detect small cancers that can't be found by CT alone.

Your health care provider may order PET/CT to clarify or check CT results. The scan will extend from the base of your skull to your knees. If PET/CT can't be done, you may get a bone scan.

Bone imaging

If initial imaging suggests a limited-stage cancer, you may undergo bone imaging.

X-rays or MRI may be used. If this imaging doesn't detect cancer, you may need a bone biopsy.

Biopsies

If imaging suggests that you may have SCLC, your health care provider will order more tests for further staging. Your health care providers need to know the correct cancer stage for treatment planning.

Pleural fluid biopsy

The lungs are covered by two layers of tissue called pleura. There is fluid between the two layers. Some people with lung cancer have an excess of this fluid, which is called pleural effusion.

If you have pleural effusion, a biopsy is needed. A needle biopsy, called a thoracentesis, may be used to remove some of the fluid for testing. If results are unclear, a thoracoscopy may be done next. A thoracoscopy involves making small openings called ports into your chest. Small tools are inserted through the ports to remove tissue.

Thoracoscopy is also called video-assisted thoracoscopic surgery (VATS).

Bone marrow biopsy

Most bones have a soft center called marrow. Your blood tests may suggest that the cancer has spread to your bone marrow. In this case, tests of bone marrow are needed.

There are two methods of removing bone marrow, which may be done at the same time.

- A bone marrow biopsy removes a core of bone and soft bone marrow.
- A bone marrow aspiration removes liquid bone marrow.

Lymph node biopsy

The space between your lungs is called the mediastinum. This space has many disease-fighting clumps of tissue called lymph nodes. Lung cancer tends to spread from inside the lung to these nodes.

If stage 1 or 2A cancer may be treated with surgery, a biopsy of mediastinal nodes is needed. The biopsy is used to confirm that there is no cancer in these lymph nodes. These nodes may be biopsied by mediastinoscopy, mediastinotomy, endobronchial or esophageal ultrasound-guided biopsy, or VATS.

Staging biopsies for limited-stage cancer

If the cancer may be limited stage, a biopsy may be needed. The biopsy will confirm that the cancer has not spread outside the lung. The image on the top shows a biopsy of bone and bone marrow. The image on the bottom shows a procedure called an endoscopic ultrasound-guided biopsy. Tissue can be removed with the scoping tool that is guided down the throat.

Bone Marrow Aspiration and Biopsy

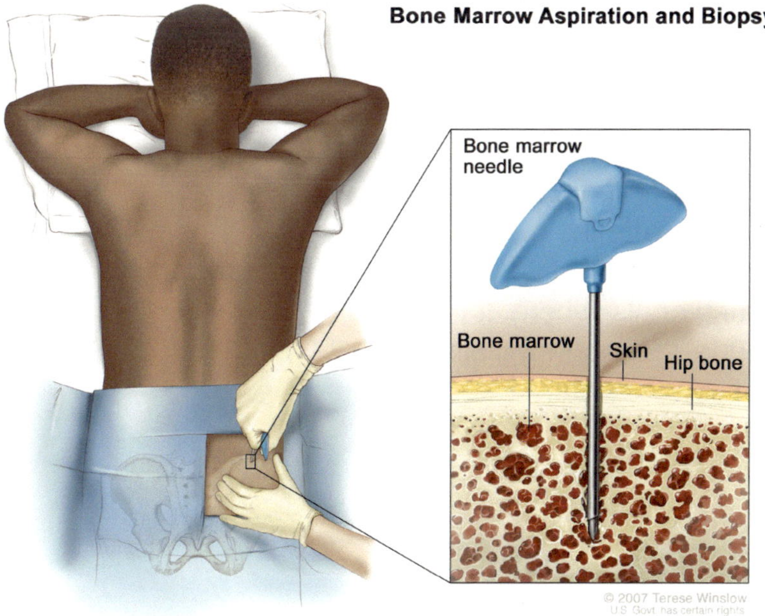

Endoscopic Ultrasound (EUS)

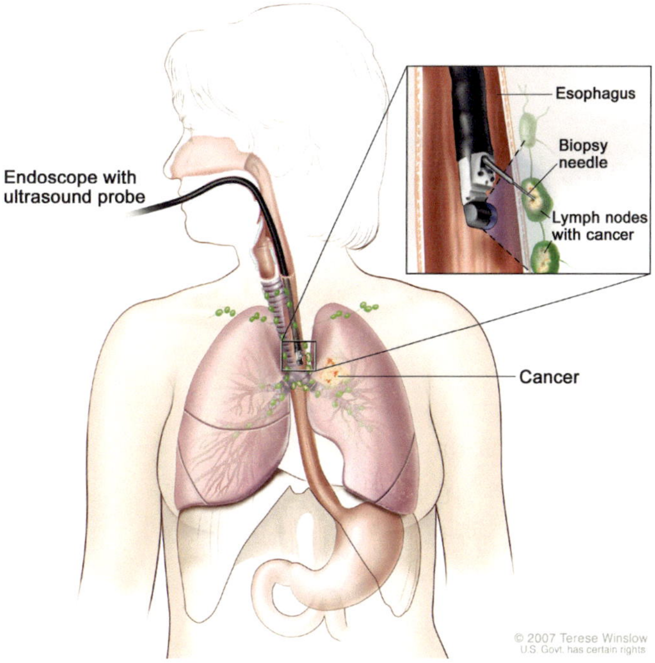

Cancer cell tests

Body tissue that is removed during biopsy or surgery will be sent to a lab for testing. A pathologist will examine and test the samples.

Pathologists are health care providers who are experts in tissue and cells and diagnosing cancer.

Pathology review

Pathologists study tissue with a microscope to classify the disease. This is called histologic typing. The pathologist will write the results in a report. The pathology report will state if the cancer started in the lung or elsewhere. If the cancer started in the lung, the report will also list the type of lung cancer.

Pathologists study tissue for cancer staging. Before treatment, you may have tissue samples removed other than the lung tumor. An example is lymph nodes. Lymph nodes are also removed during surgical treatment. The pathologist will study the tissue for cancer cells. Health care providers use pathology results to stage the cancer.

Pathologists study tissue to assess treatment results. If you have surgery for treatment, the pathologist will study the edge of the removed tissue for cancer cells. Health care providers use the pathology results to plan the next steps of treatment.

All pathology reports will be sent to your cancer health care providers. Before treatment, you may have tissue samples removed other than from the lung.

Ask for a copy of the pathology reports. Your health care providers will review the results with you. Take notes and ask questions. Your health care providers will use the reports to plan your treatment.

Key points

- Your health care providers will order tests to learn about your health and cancer. They will make a treatment plan for you based on the results.
- Your health care providers will examine your body for signs of disease. The exam will include touching parts of your body to see if anything feels abnormal.
- Your health care providers will rate your ability to do day-to-day activities to decide your treatment options.
- Your health care providers will order blood tests. Blood tests are used to assess general health and where the cancer may have spread.
- CT and MRI scans are first used to look for cancer spread. PET/CT may help detect cancer not found by CT alone. If cancer isn't detected in bone by initial imaging, you may get x-rays or MRI of bones.
- If imaging doesn't detect cancer outside the lungs, you may get biopsies of pleural fluid, bone marrow, or lymph nodes between the lungs.
- For limited-stage cancer, your lungs will be tested to assess if surgery or radiation therapy are options.

“

Take care of your mental and emotional self. Get organized and be prepared to be your own advocate. Ask the hard questions. Start a notebook and take it to all appointments to note what is said."

4

Initial treatment

Initial treatment of small cell lung cancer has good results for many people. Treatment options are based on the cancer stage and other factors. Discuss with your care team which options in this chapter are right for you.

Advances in treatment

The classic treatment for small cell lung cancer (SCLC) is chemotherapy. Chemotherapy is a type of whole-body (systemic) therapy. It travels in the bloodstream to cancer cells. It works by stopping cancer cells from making more cancer cells.

Researchers have studied which chemotherapy drugs work best. Initial treatments include two chemotherapy drugs, one of which is made with platinum. This is called platinum-doublet chemotherapy.

Stage-based treatment

Cancer staging has changed the practice of treatment. Care teams plan more precise treatment when using cancer stages.

- Limited stage includes cancers that are stage 1 to 3 and can be treated with radiation and chemotherapy with a goal of curing the disease.
- Extensive stage includes any cancers, including stage 4, that can't be treated with high radiation doses, but can be treated with chemotherapy and immunotherapy. Radiation in this stage can't cure the cancer.

Systemic therapy

Systemic therapy for lung cancer includes chemotherapy and immunotherapy. Most often, chemotherapy is a liquid that is slowly injected into a vein, called an infusion, but sometimes it is a pill. Immunotherapy is only given by infusion. Systemic therapy is given in cycles of treatment days followed by rest days. Cycles give your body a chance to recover after receiving treatment.

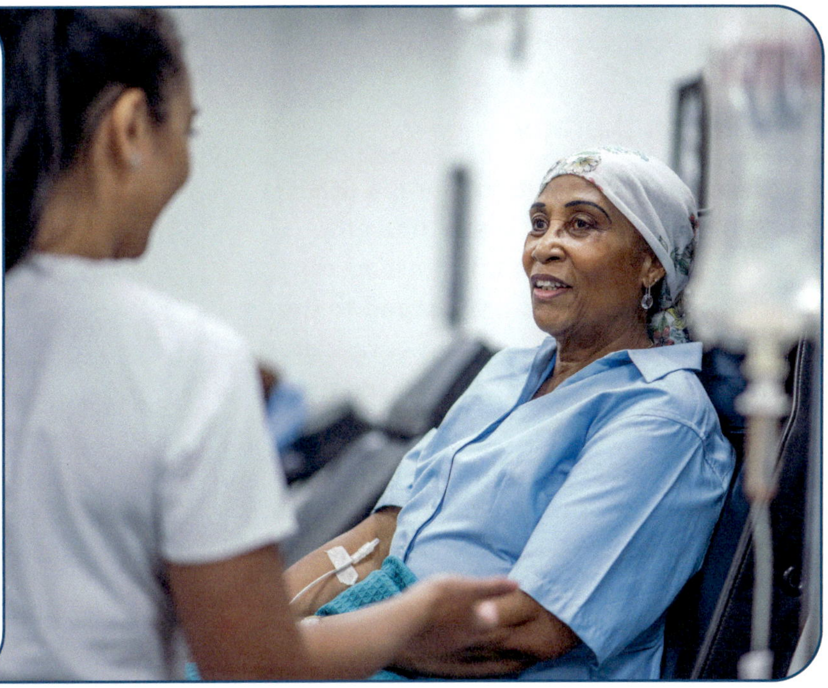

Radiation therapy uses high-energy x-rays to treat lung cancer. It damages cancer cells. The cancer cells either die or stop making new cancer cells. Radiation therapy is a local treatment. Modern techniques shape the radiation dose to the tumor to spare healthy tissue.

Radiation therapy has a role in all stages of lung cancer. It is mainly used to attempt to cure limited-stage cancer, and to reduce certain symptoms caused by extensive-stage cancer. Surgery is another local treatment used to cure some limited-stage cancers.

"Your medical team is your greatest asset and friend(s), especially the nurses. They are all highly skilled and sincerely dedicated to help you however they can."

New treatments

Treatment of extensive-stage cancer has improved in recent years. One advance is the addition of immunotherapy. Immunotherapy is a systemic therapy like chemotherapy. It uses the body's defense against disease, called the immune system, to kill cancer cells.

Radiation therapy

External beam radiation therapy (EBRT) is the most common method used for treatment. A large machine makes radiation beams that are shaped to the form of the tumor. The highest radiation dose is aimed at the cancer. A much lower dose is given to nearby tissue. You will not feel anything during the treatment session. Treatment does not make you radioactive.

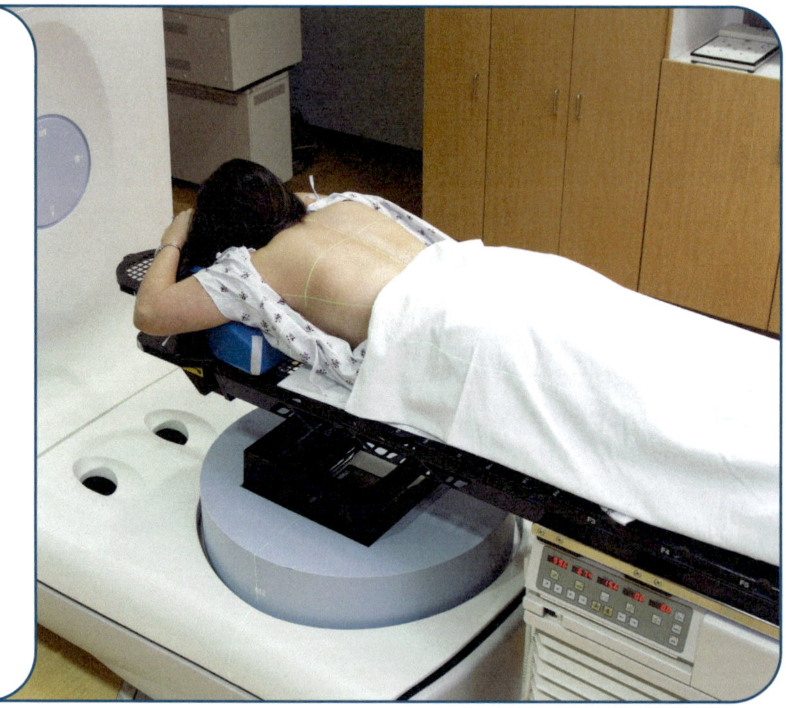

Options for limited-stage cancer

The goal of initial treatment for limited-stage cancer is to cure the cancer. Chemotherapy is often used with local treatment. Options for initial treatment of limited-stage cancer are listed in **Guide 3.**

Most people receive 4 cycles of chemotherapy. There are typically 21 to 28 days in a cycle. Limited-stage cancer is treated with either cisplatin and etoposide or carboplatin and etoposide. Immunotherapy has been recently found to be useful after the initial chemoradiation treatment has been delivered.

Chemoradiation

Most limited-stage cancers are treated with both chemotherapy and radiation therapy. This combined treatment is called chemoradiation.

Concurrent chemoradiation is the use of both treatments at the same time. Radiation therapy should be started during the first or

Guide 3
Options for initial treatment of limited-stage SCLC

Cancer stages 1A, 1B, and 2A	• Concurrent chemoradiation
	• Lobectomy and either lymph node dissection or sampling followed by:
	  • Chemotherapy if no cancer is found in lymph nodes
	  • Chemotherapy, concurrent chemoradiation, or sequential chemoradiation if cancer is found only in lymph nodes within the lungs
	  • Concurrent or sequential chemoradiation if cancer is found in lymph nodes between the lungs
	• Radiation followed by chemotherapy

Cancer stages 2B, 3A, 3B, and 3C	**Performance score of 0, 1, or 2** • Concurrent chemoradiation
	Performance score of 3 or 4 caused by the cancer • Chemotherapy • Concurrent chemoradiation • Sequential chemoradiation
	Performance score of 3 or 4 not due to the cancer • Individualized treatment including supportive care

second cycle of chemotherapy. Sequential chemoradiation is the use of one treatment followed by the other. There are advantages and disadvantages and you will have a conversation about the risks and benefits of each approach.

Performance status is your ability to do day-to-day activities. Diseases like cancer can limit what you can do. Health care providers use performance status to decide which treatments may be safe for you. Lower performance scores represent a better ability to do self-care. Chemoradiation may not be an option when scores are high.

Surgery

Some people with limited stage 1 or 2A may be able to have surgery. There must be no cancer in the biopsy samples of the lymph nodes between the lungs. The lung tumor is often removed during a surgery called a lobectomy. If cancer is only in one lobe of the

Lobectomy

Lobectomy is a type of surgery that removes an entire lobe of the lung. The surgery can be done with one of two methods. The classic method is thoracotomy. This surgery removes tissue through a large opening in the chest.

Thoracoscopy is a newer method. A small camera and surgical tools are inserted through small openings. Thoracoscopy can be done with or without help from a robot. Thoracoscopy is also called video-assisted thoracoscopic surgery (VATS).

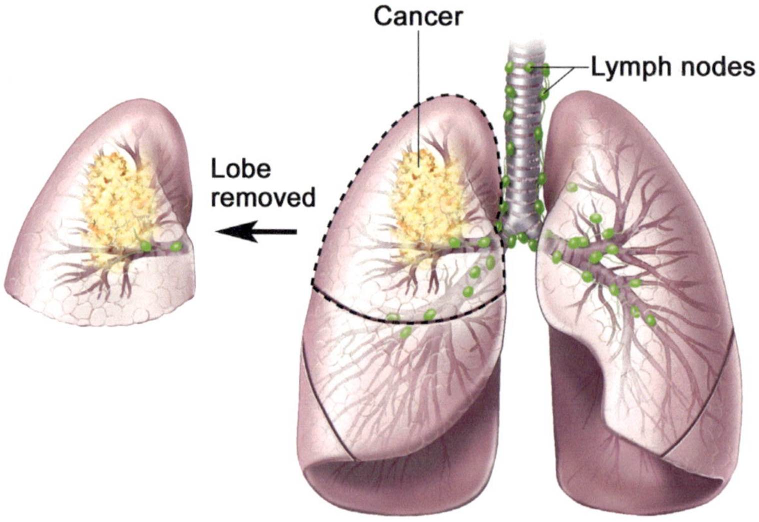

lungs, a lobectomy removes an entire lobe of the lung.

During surgery, lymph nodes will also be removed to test them for cancer. A lymph node sampling removes some nodes in and between the lungs.

A lymph node dissection removes as many nodes as possible from the lung and between the lungs.

Some hard-to-detect cancer cells are almost always left behind even after surgery. So you will receive chemotherapy after surgery to treat any remaining cancer cells. Treatment for this purpose is called adjuvant therapy.

Radiation therapy to the chest may also be received at the same time or back-to-back. It may improve results if cancer is in mediastinal lymph nodes.

SABR

Stereotactic ablative radiotherapy (SABR) may be an option for people who don't have surgery. SABR is also called stereotactic body radiation therapy (SBRT).

SABR delivers a high radiation dose to a precise area. Afterward, you will receive systemic therapy to treat any remaining cancer cells. Treatment for this purpose is called adjuvant therapy.

> "Please allow yourself to accept hard days, difficult moments, or disappointments. Speaking with a behavioral health specialist can help you prepare for the emotional changes that you may face."

Options for extensive-stage cancer

The goals of treatment for extensive-stage cancer are to control symptoms and to prolong life. Systemic therapy is the main treatment.

You will likely receive four 21-day cycles of chemoimmunotherapy, but some people receive up to six cycles. This is often followed by immunotherapy alone.

Options for initial systemic therapy of extensive-stage cancer are listed in **Guide 4.**

Chemoimmunotherapy

The preferred treatment for extensive-stage cancer is chemoimmunotherapy. Platinum-doublet chemotherapy is given with an immunotherapy medicine called an immune checkpoint inhibitor. Immune checkpoint inhibitors enable immune cells called T cells to attack cancer cells.

After chemoimmunotherapy, you may stay on the checkpoint inhibitor if treatment results show the tumor is stable/not getting worse, not growing, and has not spread. This is called maintenance. The goal of maintenance treatment is to prolong good treatment results.

- Maintenance atezolizumab is received every 21 or 28 days depending on the regimen.
- Maintenance durvalumab is received every 28 days. Often, people get infusions to delay the worsening of cancer.

Chemotherapy

Not all lung cancers should be treated with immunotherapy. Immunotherapy may not be safe if you're too sick. Also, it may impair your

Guide 4
Options for initial systemic therapy of extensive-stage SCLC

Preferred options	• Carboplatin, etoposide, and atezolizumab followed by maintenance atezolizumab • Carboplatin, etoposide, and durvalumab followed by maintenance durvalumab • Cisplatin, etoposide, and durvalumab followed by maintenance durvalumab
Other options	• Carboplatin and etoposide • Cisplatin and etoposide
Sometimes useful	• Carboplatin and irinotecan • Cisplatin and irinotecan

immune system if you have an autoimmune disease.

Autoimmune diseases include Crohn's disease, ulcerative colitis, and lupus. When immunotherapy is not an option, you may receive only chemotherapy.

Radiation therapy

In addition to systemic therapy, you may get radiation therapy. Radiation therapy can reduce (palliate) symptoms caused by lung cancer, such as:

- Swelling caused by the cancer blocking a vein called the superior vena cava
- Bone pain due to the cancer damaging bone
- Back pain from the cancer pressing on the spinal cord
- Trouble breathing due to the cancer blocking airways
- Headaches from lung cancer in the brain

Treatment of the brain usually involves radiation to the entire brain, which is called whole-brain radiation therapy (WBRT).

Some people can receive a high radiation dose just to the affected area of the brain.

When lung cancer has spread to the brain, radiation therapy is sometimes received before it causes symptoms.

During systemic therapy, your health care provider will assess the status of the cancer. After every 2 cycles, you will get either MRI or CT scans of the brain. Contrast should be used with CT. If the cancer worsens, radiation therapy of the brain will be started.

What are the techniques of EBRT?

External beam radiation therapy (EBRT) is the most common radiaiton treatment method for SCLC. It may be delivered by one of several techniques:

- Intensity-modulated radiation therapy (IMRT) delivers x-ray beams that closely match the target's shape and spare more normal tissue.
- Volumetric modulated arc therapy (VMAT) delivers IMRT in an arc shape around the tumor.
- Three-dimensional conformal radiation therapy (3D-CRT) delivers an x-ray beam that matches the shape of the target but may not be as focused as IMRT.

Cancer treatment with IMRT, VMAT, and 3D-CRT is typically delivered daily Monday through Friday and finishes in about 6 weeks. Radiation therapy for symptoms is finished in 10 or fewer sessions. Newer techniques for small tumors are also finished in a shorter amount of time:

- Stereotactic radiosurgery (SRS) treats small tumors with very precise, high-dose x-ray beams.
- When SRS is used to treat tumors not in the brain or spine, it is called stereotactic ablative radiotherapy (SABR).

SRS is finished in one or a few sessions. SABR is given two to three times per week. Treatment is finished in about 1½ weeks.

Treatment response

A treatment response is how well someone improves with treatment and how much the cancer shrinks. Many SCLCs respond strongly to initial treatment. The timing of assessing the treatment response differs between treatment types and the cancer stage.

For limited-stage cancer, the treatment response should be assessed:

- After concurrent chemoradiation
- During sequential chemoradiation and after treatment
- During systemic therapy (without radiation therapy) and after treatment

For extensive-stage cancer, the treatment response should be assessed:

- After every 2 to 3 cycles of systemic therapy and after treatment

To assess the treatment response, you will repeat some blood and imaging tests.

Your health care providers will assess the treatment response based on test results. There are 4 possible treatment responses:

- Complete remission is the most effective result. There are no signs of cancer.
- Partial remission means that the tumors have shrunk, and blood results are returning to normal.
- Stable disease is less than a partial remission. The cancer is not getting worse.
- Progressive disease is the cancer getting worse. Treatment options for progressive disease are the same as for relapse listed in Chapter 5.

Additional radiation therapy

After treatment response is assessed, you may receive radiation therapy. Prophylactic cranial irradiation (PCI) is an option for limited- and extensive-stage cancer.

Some people with extensive-stage cancer may also receive radiation therapy to the chest.

Prophylactic cranial irradiation

PCI is a low dose of radiation to the brain to prevent the cancer from growing in the brain. Cancer researchers are still learning which patients benefit the most from this treatment.

It may be an option if any of these conditions apply to you:

- A complete or partial remission of cancer was achieved.
- There are no signs or symptoms of lung cancer in the brain.
- You do not have problems with things like your memory.
- Your health doesn't largely limit your day-to-day activities.

For some limited-stage cancers, PCI can prevent lung cancer tumors in the brain and prolong life. For extensive-stage cancer, PCI can prevent or delay lung cancer from forming tumors in the brain.

The decision whether to pursue this should be individualized to each person after a discussion of the pros and cons in that specific scenario. An alternative to this type of treatment is to hold off on treatment, but obtain a CT or MRI of the brain every 6 months.

Radiation therapy to the chest

If systemic therapy achieved complete or partial remission of extensive-stage cancer, then chest radiation can be used to treat any cancer that remains Treatment for this purpose is called consolidation therapy.

Chest radiation may prevent the cancer from returning in the chest and prolong life.

"No matter what I look like on the outside, it's not who I am on the inside. Stay positive and stay strong."

Clinical trials

Therapy may also be available as part of a clinical trial. A clinical trial is a type of medical research study and a vital way to assess new treatment methods.

After being developed and tested in a laboratory, potential new ways of fighting cancer need to be studied in people. If found to be safe and effective in a clinical trial, a drug, device, or treatment approach may be approved by the FDA.

Everyone with cancer should carefully consider all of the treatment options available for their cancer type, including standard treatments and clinical trials. Talk to your health care provider about whether a clinical trial may make sense for you.

Phases

Most cancer clinical trials focus on treatment. Treatment trials are done in phases.

- **Phase 1** trials study the dose, safety, and side effects of an investigational drug or treatment approach. They also look for early signs that the drug or approach is helpful.
- **Phase 2** trials study how well the drug or approach works against a specific type of cancer.
- **Phase 3** trials test the drug or approach against a standard treatment. If the results are good, it may be approved by the FDA.
- **Phase 4** trials study the long-term safety and benefit of an FDA-approved treatment.

Who can enroll?

Every clinical trial has rules for joining, called eligibility criteria. The rules may be about age, cancer type and stage, treatment history, or general health. These requirements ensure that participants are alike in specific ways in order to compare how they respond to a specific treatment.

Informed consent

Clinical trials are managed by a group of experts called a research team. The research team will review the study with you in detail, including its purpose and the risks and benefits of joining. All of this information is also provided in an informed consent form. This agreement confirms that you've been fully told about your part in the trial. Read the form carefully and ask questions before signing it. Take time to discuss with family, friends, or others whom you trust. Keep in mind that you can leave and seek treatment outside of the clinical trial at any time.

Start the conversation

Don't wait for your health care provider to bring up clinical trials. Start the conversation and learn about all of your treatment options. Ask if a clinical trial is available for your situation. If you find a study that you may be eligible for, ask your treatment team if you meet the requirements. If you have already started standard treatment, you may not be eligible for certain clinical trials. Try not to be discouraged if you cannot join. New clinical trials are always becoming available.

Frequently asked questions

There are many myths and misconceptions surrounding clinical trials. The possible benefits and risks are not well understood by many with cancer.

Will I get a placebo?

Placebos (inactive versions of real medicines) are almost never used alone in cancer clinical trials. It's common to receive either a placebo with a standard treatment or a new drug with a standard treatment. You'll be informed if a placebo is part of a clinical trial before you enroll.

Do I have to pay to be in a clinical trial?

There's no fee to enroll in a clinical trial. The study sponsor pays for research-related costs, including the study drug. You may, however, have costs indirectly related to the trial, such as the cost of transportation or childcare due to extra appointments. During the trial, you'll continue to receive standard cancer care. This care is billed to—and often covered by—insurance. You're responsible for copays and any costs for this care that aren't covered by your insurance.

Finding a clinical trial

In the United States

NCCN Cancer Centers
NCCN.org/cancercenters

The National Cancer Institute (NCI)
cancer.gov/about-cancer/treatment/clinical-trials/search

Worldwide

The U.S. National Library of Medicine (NLM)
clinicaltrials.gov

Need help finding a clinical trial?

NCI's Cancer Information Service (CIS)
1.800.4.CANCER (1.800.422.6237)
cancer.gov/contact

Supportive care

Supportive care aims to improve your quality of life. It's also sometimes called palliative care, but it is more than that. Supportive care is important for everyone and is encouraged for people at all stages of cancer, not just people at the end of life.

Supportive care can address many needs. It includes care for health problems caused by cancer or cancer treatment. You can get help with making treatment decisions. You can get help with the coordination of care between health providers.

Your supportive care specialist will work with your oncologists to provide you with the best care. Other specialists that may be involved in your care include:

- Respiratory therapists
- Rehabilitation specialists
- Registered dieticians
- Social workers

Side effects

All cancer treatments can cause unwanted health issues. Such health issues are called side effects. Some side effects may be harmful to your health. Others may just be unpleasant.

Side effects depend on many factors. These factors include the treatment type, length or dose of treatment, and the person. Many effects of treatment resolve after treatment ends, such as:

- Nausea and vomiting from chemotherapy
- Side effects such as a fever, rash, or inflammation in vital organs (such as inflammation in the lungs, liver, or thyroid) from an immune checkpoint inhibitor
- Fatigue and skin changes from radiation therapy
- Pain and swelling from surgery

Long-term effects start during treatment and persist after treatment is done. Less often, effects start long after treatment has ended. Ask your treatment team for a complete list of side effects of your treatments.

Also, tell your treatment team about any new or worse symptoms you get. There may be ways to help you feel better. There are also ways to prevent some side effects. An example is a medication called memantine that helps to prevent a decline in thinking skills after PCI.

Key points

- Advances in lung cancer treatment have been made using staging systems and through the use of new medicines.
- Options for initial treatment of limited-stage cancer include chemoradiation, stereotactic ablative radiotherapy (SABR), and surgery. After initial treatment, you may receive chemotherapy with or without radiation therapy.
- Options for initial treatment of extensive-stage cancer are chemoimmunotherapy and chemotherapy. Some people receive radiation therapy to prevent or relieve symptoms caused by the cancer.
- The response to treatment will be assessed. You may get radiation therapy to the brain or chest if the right conditions are met.
- New ways of fighting cancer are studied among people in clinical trials. A clinical trial may be an option in addition to standard treatment.
- Supportive care aims to improve your quality of life. A main goal of supportive care is to relieve symptoms caused by cancer treatment.

Supportive care is for everyone, not just people at the end of life.

Use the resources available to you and care for your whole self, not just your cancer.

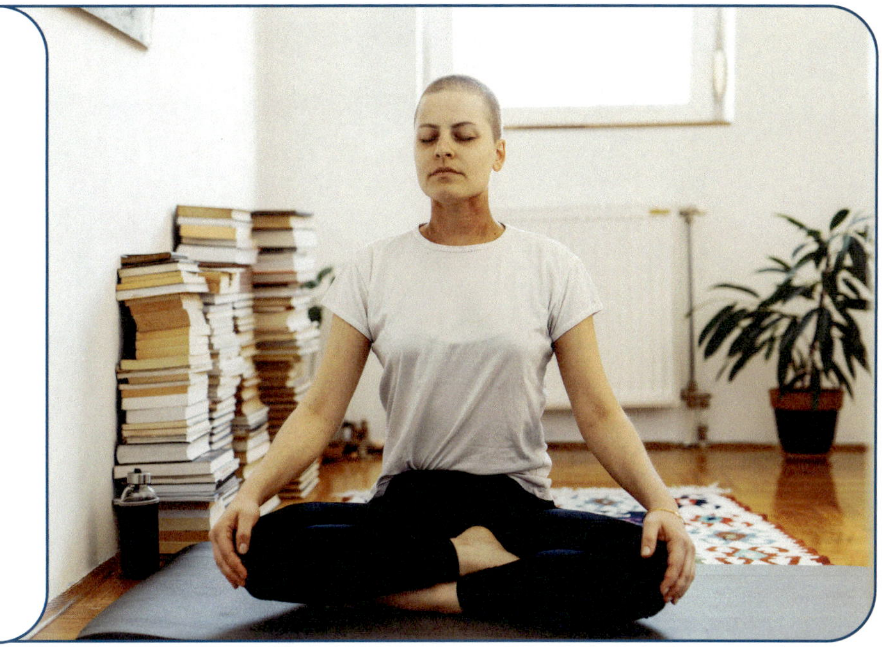

5

Surveillance and subsequent treatment

Your cancer health care providers will give you a care plan at the end of initial treatment. This care plan will include follow-up visits, possible late effects, and goals for healthy living. This chapter explains more about what comes after treatment.

Follow-up visits

You will meet with your cancer care team often after treatment ends. It's very important to monitor for the return or worsening of the cancer. The return of cancer is called a relapse or recurrence. Routine testing for cancer relapse is called surveillance. It may find cancer early and allow for timely treatment.

At follow-up visits, your health care provider will perform a medical history and a physical exam. Blood tests may be ordered if needed. **See Guide 5** for a schedule of visits with your cancer care provider.

Guide 5
How often to see your cancer health care provider after treatment

Limited-stage cancer	During first year	Every 3 months
	During second year	Every 3 months
	During third year	Every 6 months
	During fourth year	Once a year
	During fifth year	Once a year
	During sixth year and beyond	Once a year
Extensive-stage cancer	During first year	Every 2 months
	During second year	Every 3 to 4 months
	During third year	Every 3 to 4 months
	During fourth year	Every 6 months
	During fifth year	Every 6 months
	During sixth year and beyond	Once a year

Imaging

Your health care provider will order a CT, a machine that you lie inside that takes many x-rays at once. It may detect a relapse. CT of your chest, abdomen, and, sometimes, pelvis may be done every 2 to 6 months. If a new lung nodule is detected, more testing will be needed to confirm if it is cancer.

An MRI (another machine you lie inside that takes pictures using magnets) may show small brain tumors that aren't causing symptoms. Contrast, a liquid injected into your vein that shows blood vessels better, should be used.

If MRI can't be done, you may get a CT with contrast of your head. Brain MRI or CT of the head should be done every 3 to 4 months during the first year after treatment. During the second year, this imaging should be done every 6 months.

Managing side effects

All cancer treatments can cause health issues called side effects. Many effects of treatment quickly resolve after treatment ends. An example is nausea and vomiting. Long-term effects start during treatment and persist after treatment is done. Sometimes (but less often), effects start long after treatment is over. These are called late effects.

During follow-up visits, your health care providers will assess for side effects. They will provide treatment for side effects as needed.

Read about common effects in *NCCN Guidelines for Patients: Survivorship Care for Cancer-Related Late and Long-Term Effects,* available at NCCN.org/patientguidelines and on the NCCN Patient Guides for Cancer app.

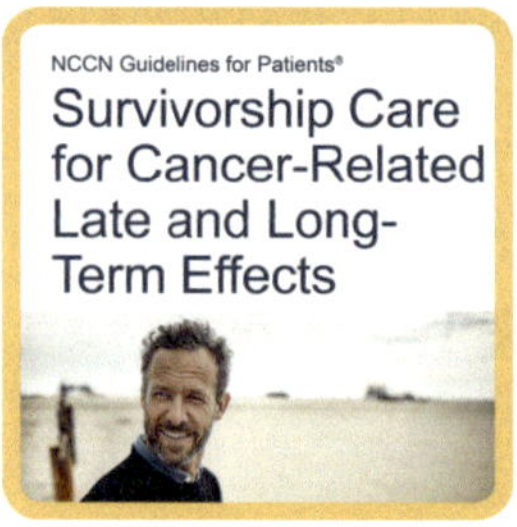

Healthy living

Another part of follow-up care is to prevent diseases. Such care can include getting immunization shots for the flu, herpes, shingles, and other diseases. Dental cleaning and regular exams can prevent disease, too.

Other common goals for healthy living include:

- Seeing a primary care provider regularly
- Being physically active and avoiding inactivity
- Eating healthful foods
- Limiting or avoiding drinking alcohol
- Achieving and maintaining a healthy body weight
- Not using tobacco
- Avoiding infections and getting vaccines as recommended

Read about preventing poor health in *NCCN Guidelines for Patients: Survivorship Care for Healthy Living*, available at NCCN.org/patientguidelines and on the NCCN Patient Guides for Cancer app.

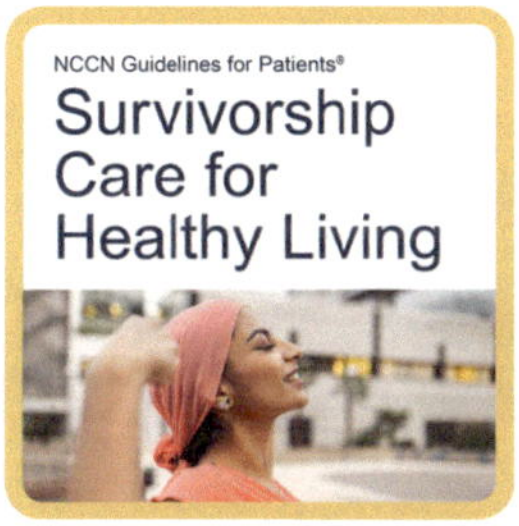

If you have a high risk for certain cancers, you may enroll in a screening program. Cancer screening is routine testing for common cancers before cancer symptoms start.

You may be screened for:

- Prostate cancer
- Breast cancer
- Cervical cancer
- Colorectal cancer
- Skin cancer

"Ask your oncologist for a list of possible side effects right before each treatment. Track your side effects and report them to your doctor."

Treatment for relapse

SCLC relapses in most people. Health care providers use performance status to decide which treatments may be safe for you.

Performance status is your ability to do day-to-day activities.

Performance status consists of five scores ranging from 0 to 5. Lower scores represent a better ability to do self-care.

Guide 6
Treatment options for relapse

Preferred options	Topotecan
	Lurbinectedin
	Clinical trial*
	Tarlatamab-dlle
Other options	Paclitaxel
	Docetaxel
	Irinotecan
	Temozolomide
	Cyclophosphamide, doxorubicin, and vincristine (CAV)
	Oral etoposide
	Vinorelbine
	Gemcitabine
	Nivolumab
	Pembrolizumab
	Bendamustine

* Not recommended for relapse over 6 months.

A treatment option for people with performance scores of 0 to 2 is systemic therapy. Options differ based on a relapse that occurred less or more than 6 months after systemic therapy.

Read Guide 6 for a list of treatment options for relapsed disease.

If a relapse occurs before 6 months, the preferred options are chemotherapy or a clinical trial.

If a relapse occurs after 6 months, the preferred option is the same systemic therapy you received for your initial treatment. So if chemotherapy was your initial treatment, you can have that chemotherapy again to treat a SCLC relapse.

Other options are chemotherapy and immunotherapy. Pembrolizumab (Keytruda) and nivolumab (Opdivo) are immune checkpoint inhibitors.

If treatment may do more harm than good, supportive care is an option. Supportive care aims to improve quality of life. It's also called palliative care. Supportive care may include radiation therapy for the relief of symptoms.

Key points

- Your cancer care providers will monitor for a return of lung cancer. Regular testing for cancer relapse is called surveillance.
- Some side effects of treatment are long-term or may appear years later.
- Tell your care team about any new or worse symptoms. There are ways to prevent or treat most side effects.
- If you have a high risk for certain cancers, you may enroll in a screening program.
- Treatment for a relapse includes chemotherapy, immunotherapy, and clinical trials. If treatment may do more harm than good, supportive care to improve your quality of life is an option.

6

Making treatment decisions

It is important to be comfortable with the cancer treatment you choose. This choice starts with having an open and honest conversation with your care team.

It's your choice

In shared decision-making, you and your care team share information, discuss the options, and agree on a treatment plan. It starts with an open and honest conversation between you and your team.

Treatment decisions are very personal. What is important to you may not be important to someone else. Some things that may play a role in your decision-making:

- What you want and how that might differ from what others want
- Your religious and spiritual beliefs
- Your feelings about certain treatments
- Your feelings about pain or side effects
- Cost of treatment, travel to treatment centers, and time away from school or work
- Quality of life and length of life
- How active you are and the activities that are important to you

Think about what you want from treatment. Discuss openly the risks and benefits of specific treatments and procedures. Weigh options and share concerns with your care team. If you take the time to build a relationship with your team, it will help you feel supported when considering options and making treatment decisions.

Second opinion

It is normal to want to start treatment as soon as possible. While cancer should not be ignored, there is time to have another care provider review your test results and suggest a treatment plan. This is called getting a second opinion, and it's a normal part of cancer care. Even doctors get second opinions!

Things you can do to prepare:

- Check with your insurance company about its rules on second opinions. There may be out-of-pocket costs to see doctors who are not part of your insurance plan.
- Make plans to have copies of all your records sent to the doctor you will see for your second opinion.

Support groups

Many people diagnosed with cancer find support groups to be helpful. Support groups often include people at different stages of treatment. Some people may be newly diagnosed, while others may be finished with treatment. If your hospital or community doesn't have support groups for people with cancer, check out the websites listed in this book.

Questions to ask

Possible questions to ask your care team are listed on the following pages. Feel free to use these or come up with your own.

Questions about cancer testing

1. What tests will I have?
2. Do the tests have any risks?
3. Will my insurance pay for all of the tests you are recommending?
4. Do I need to do anything to prepare for testing?
5. Should I bring someone with me to the appointments?
6. Where do I go for testing, and how long will it take?
7. If any of the tests will hurt, what will you do to make me comfortable?
8. How soon will I know the results and who will explain them to me?
9. How can I get a copy of the pathology report and other test results?
10. Is there an online portal with my test results?

Questions about treatment options

1. What are my treatment options?
2. Is a clinical trial an option for me?
3. What will happen if I do nothing?
4. Are you suggesting options other than what NCCN recommends? If yes, why?
5. How do my age, sex, overall health, and other factors affect my options?
6. What if I am pregnant, or planning to become pregnant?
7. Does any option offer a cure or long-term cancer control?
8. What are the side effects of the treatments?
9. How do I get a second opinion?
10. How long do I have to decide about treatment, and is there a social worker or someone who can help me decide?

Questions about resources and support

1. Who can I talk to about help with housing, food, and other basic needs?
2. What assistance is available for transportation, childcare, and home care?
3. Who can tell me what my options for health insurance are and assist me with applying for insurance coverage?
4. How much will I have to pay for my treatment? What help is available to pay for medicines and other treatment?
5. Who can help me with my concerns about work or school?
6. How can I connect with others and build a support system?
7. Who can I talk to if I don't feel safe at home, at work, or in my neighborhood?

Questions about what to expect

1. Does this hospital or cancer center offer the best treatment for me?
2. Do I have a choice of when to begin treatment?
3. How long will treatment last?
4. Will my insurance cover the treatment you're recommending?
5. Are there any programs to help pay for treatment?
6. What supportive care and services are available to me and my caregivers?
7. Who should I contact with questions or concerns if the office is closed?
8. How will you know if treatment is working?
9. What are the chances of the cancer worsening or returning?
10. What follow-up care is needed after treatment?

Questions about side effects

1. What are the possible complications and side effects of treatment?
2. Does the cancer itself cause any side effects?
3. Which side effects are most common and how long do they usually last?
4. Which side effects are serious or life-threatening?
5. Are there any long-term or permanent side effects?
6. What symptoms should I report right away, and who do I contact?
7. What can I do to prevent or relieve the side effects of treatment?
8. Do any medications worsen side effects?
9. Do any side effects lessen or worsen in severity over time?
10. Will you stop or change treatment if there are serious side effects?

Questions about clinical trials

1. Do you recommend that I consider a clinical trial for treatment?
2. How do I find clinical trials that I can participate in?
3. What are the treatments used in the clinical trial?
4. Has the treatment been used for other types of cancer?
5. What are the risks and benefits of this treatment?
6. What side effects should I expect and how will they be managed?
7. How long will I be in the clinical trial?
8. Will I be able to get other treatment if this doesn't work?
9. How will you know if the treatment is working?
10. Will the clinical trial cost me anything?

Questions about your care team's experience

1. Are you board certified? If yes, in what area?
2. What is your experience as well as your team's experience with treating the type of cancer I have?
3. How many patients like me (of the same age, gender, race) have you treated?
4. Will you be consulting with experts to discuss my care? Whom will you consult?
5. Is this treatment (or procedure) a major part of your practice? How often have you done this treatment (or procedure) in the last year?
6. How many of your patients have had complications? What were the complications?

Resources

American Lung Association
lung.org/lung-health-diseases/lung-disease-lookup/lung-cancer

Cancer*Care*
Cancercare.org

Caring Ambassadors Program, Inc.
LungCancerCAP.org

Free Me from Lung Cancer
freemefromlungcancer.org

GO2 Foundation for Lung Cancer
go2foundation.org

Imerman Angels
Imermanangels.org

LiveLung (Dusty Joy Foundation)
dustyjoy.org

LUNGevity
Lungevity.org

Lung Cancer Action Network (LungCAN)
lungcan.org

Lung Cancer Research Foundation
lungcancerresearchfoundation.org

National Coalition for Cancer Survivorship
canceradvocacy.org

Triage Cancer
triagecancer.org

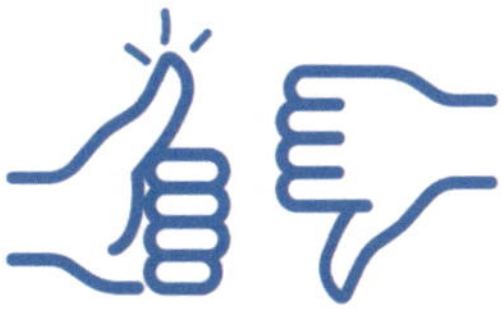

Let us know what you think!

Please take a moment to complete an online survey about the NCCN Guidelines for Patients.

NCCN.org/patients/response

Words to know

alveoli
The tiny sacs in the lungs where gases are transferred in and out of the blood.

biomarker testing
Tests of any molecule in your body that can be measured to assess your health.

biopsy
A procedure that removes fluid or tissue samples to be tested for a disease.

blood urea nitrogen (BUN)
The amount of urea nitrogen—a waste product—in blood.

board certified
A status for health care providers who finished training in a specialized field of medicine.

body plethysmograph
A test of how much air is in your lungs after inhaling or exhaling.

bronchi
The two airways extending from the windpipe into the lungs.

bronchioli
Small airways within the lungs.

bronchus
One of the two main airways that extends into the lungs.

cancer stage
A rating of the outlook of a cancer based on its growth and spread.

carcinoma
A cancer of cells that line the inner or outer surfaces of the body.

chemoradiation
A cancer treatment with both cell-killing drugs and high-energy rays.

chemotherapy
Cancer drugs that stop the cell life cycle so cells don't increase in number.

clinical stage
The rating of the extent of cancer before treatment is started.

clinical trial
A type of research that assesses how well health tests or treatments work in people.

complete blood count (CBC)
A lab test that measures the parts of the blood.

computed tomography (CT)
A test that uses x-rays from many angles to make a picture of the insides of the body.

contrast
A dye put into your body to make clearer pictures during imaging.

creatinine
A waste product of muscles that is filtered out of blood into urine by the kidneys.

diagnosis
An identification of an illness based on tests.

endobronchial ultrasound–guided biopsy
A procedure that removes lung tissue with a needle on an imaging device guided down the windpipe.

esophageal ultrasound–guided biopsy
A procedure that removes lung tissue with a needle on an imaging device guided down the food pipe (esophagus).

external beam radiation therapy (EBRT)
A cancer treatment with radiation delivered from a machine outside the body.

gas diffusion
A test that uses harmless gas to measure how much you can breathe out.

immunotherapy
A treatment with drugs that help the body find and destroy cancer cells.

intensity-modulated radiation therapy (IMRT)
Treatment with radiation that uses small beams of different strengths.

invasion
The growth of cancer cells from where it started into another tissue.

liver function tests
A lab test that measures chemicals made or processed by the liver.

lobe
A clearly seen division in an organ.

lobectomy
An operation that removes a whole lobe of an organ.

lymph node
A small, bean-shaped, disease-fighting structure.

magnetic resonance imaging (MRI)
A test that uses radio waves and powerful magnets to make pictures of the insides of the body.

maintenance therapy
A treatment phase that is given to prolong good treatment results.

mediastinoscopy
A procedure to do work in the chest with a device passed through a small cut in the skin.

mediastinum
The area of the chest between the lungs.

medical history
A report of all your health events and medications.

metastasis
The spread of cancer from the first tumor to a new site.

NCCN
National Comprehensive Cancer Network

neuroendocrine cell
A cell that helps heal injured cells.

non-small cell lung cancer (NSCLC)
A cancer that starts in lung cells that are not small in size.

pathologist
A health care provider who's an expert in testing cells and tissue to find disease.

patient navigator
A professional who helps people get health information and the services they need.

performance status
A rating of one's ability to do daily activities.

physical exam
A review of the body by a health expert for signs of disease.

platinum-doublet chemotherapy
A treatment with two cell-killing drugs, one of which contains the chemical platinum.

positron emission tomography (PET)
A test that uses radioactive material to see the shape and function of body parts.

positron emission tomography/computed tomography (PET/CT)
A test that uses two picture-making methods to show the shape and function of tissue.

primary tumor
The main mass of a certain type of cancer cell.

prognosis
The likely course and outcome of a disease based on tests.

prophylactic cranial irradiation (PCI)
Prevention of cancer spread to the brain using radiation therapy.

pulmonary function tests
A set of breathing tests to test the strength of the lungs.

pulmonologist
A health care provider who's an expert in lung diseases.

radiation oncologist
A health care provider who's an expert in treating cancer with radiation.

radiation therapy
A treatment that uses intense energy to kill cancer cells.

respiratory system
The group of organs that transfers gases in and out of the body.

side effect
An unhealthy or unpleasant physical or emotional response to treatment.

small cell lung cancer (SCLC)
A cancer of small, round lung cells.

spirometry
A test that uses a tube to measure how fast you breathe.

stereotactic ablative radiotherapy (SABR)
Treatment with high-dose radiation within one or a few sessions. Also called stereotactic body radiation therapy (SBRT).

stereotactic radiosurgery (SRS)
Treatment of a brain tumor with high-dose radiation within one or a few sessions.

supportive care
Health care that includes symptom relief but not cancer treatment. Also sometimes called palliative care.

surgery
An operation to remove or repair a part of the body.

thoracic radiologist
A health care provider who's an expert in reading imaging tests of the chest.

thoracic surgeon
A health care provider who's an expert in operating on organs inside the chest.

thoracoscopy
A procedure to do work in the chest with a device passed through a small cut in the skin. Also called video-assisted thoracoscopic surgery (VATS).

three-dimensional conformal radiation therapy (3D-CRT)
A treatment with radiation that uses beams matched to the shape of the tumor.

tumor, node, metastasis (TNM) system
A staging system for cancer based on three areas of cancer growth.

ultrasound
A test that uses sound waves to take pictures of the inside of the body.

Veterans Administration (VA) system
The first system created to stage small cell lung cancer.

volumetric modulated arc therapy (VMAT)
A treatment with radiation that is delivered in an arc shape around the tumor.

whole-brain radiation therapy (WBRT)
Treatment of the entire brain with radiation.

share with us.

Take our survey and help make the NCCN Guidelines for Patients better for everyone!

NCCN.org/patients/comments

NCCN Contributors

This patient guide is based on the NCCN Clinical Practice Guidelines in Oncology (NCCN Guidelines®) for Small Cell Lung Cancer, Version 3.2024. It was adapted, reviewed, and published with help from the following people:

Dorothy A. Shead, MS
Senior Director
Patient Information Operations

Tim Rinehart
Medical Writer

Susan Kidney
Senior Graphic Design Specialist

The NCCN Clinical Practice Guidelines in Oncology (NCCN Guidelines®) for Small Cell Lung Cancer, Version 3.2024 were developed by the following NCCN Panel Members:

*Apar Kishor P. Ganti, MD, Chair
Fred & Pamela Buffett Cancer Center

Billy W. Loo, Jr., MD, PhD/Vice Chair
Stanford Cancer Institute

Shahed Badiyan, MD
UT Southwestern Simmons Comprehensive Cancer Center

Michael Bassetti, MD
University of Wisconsin Carbone Cancer Center

Christine Bestvina, MD
The UChicago Medicine Comprehensive Cancer Center

Anne Chiang, MD, PhD
Yale Cancer Center/Smilow Cancer Hospital

Christopher A. D'Avella, MD
Abramson Cancer Center at the University of Pennsylvania

Megan Daly, MD
UC Davis Comprehensive Cancer Center

Afshin Dowlati, MD
Case Comprehensive Cancer Center/ University Hospitals Seidman Cancer Center and Cleveland Clinic Taussig Cancer Institute

Robert J. Downey, MD
Memorial Sloan Kettering Cancer Center

*Martin Edelman, MD
Fox Chase Cancer Center

*Charles Florsheim, JD
Patient Advocate

Kathryn A. Gold, MD
UC San Diego Moores Cancer Center

Jonathan W. Goldman, MD
UCLA Jonsson Comprehensive Cancer Center

John C. Grecula, MD
The Ohio State University Comprehensive Cancer Center - James Cancer Hospital and Solove Research Institute

Christine Hann, MD, PhD
The Sidney Kimmel Comprehensive Cancer Center at Johns Hopkins

Wade Iams, MD
Vanderbilt-Ingram Cancer Center

Maya Khalil, MD
O'Neal Comprehensive Cancer Center at UAB

Jyoti Malhotra, MD
City of Hope National Medical Center

Robert E. Merritt, MD
The Ohio State University Comprehensive Cancer Center - James Cancer Hospital and Solove Research Institute

*Nisha Mohindra, MD
Robert H. Lurie Comprehensive Cancer Center of Northwestern University

Julian R. Molina, MD, PhD
Mayo Clinic Comprehensive Cancer Center

Cesar Moran, MD
The University of Texas MD Anderson Cancer Center

Claire Mulvey, MD
UCSF Helen Diller Family Comprehensive Cancer Center

*Evan Osmundson, MD
Vanderbilt-Ingram Cancer Center

Shiven Patel, MD
Huntsman Cancer Institute at the University of Utah

Tejas Patil, MD
University of Colorado Cancer Center

Chinh Phan, DO
UC Davis Comprehensive Cancer Center

Saraswati Pokharel, MD
Roswell Park Comprehensive Cancer Center

Sonam Puri, MD
Huntsman Cancer Institute at the University of Utah

*Angel Qin, MD
University of Michigan Rogel Cancer Center

Jacob Sands, MD
Dana Farber/Brigham and Women's Cancer Center

*Rafael Santana-Davila, MD
Fred Hutchinson Cancer Center

Michael Shafique, MD
Moffitt Cancer Center

*Misty Shields, MD, PhD
Indiana University Melvin and Bren Simon Comprehensive Cancer Center

Tina Tailor, MD
Duke Cancer Institute

*Saiama N. Waqar, MD
Siteman Cancer Center at Barnes-Jewish Hospital and Washington University School of Medicine

NCCN

Carly J. Cassara, MSc
Swathi Ramakrishnan, PhD

* Reviewed this patient guide. For disclosures, visit NCCN.org/disclosures.

NCCN Cancer Centers

Abramson Cancer Center
at the University of Pennsylvania
Philadelphia, Pennsylvania
800.789.7366 • *pennmedicine.org/cancer*

Case Comprehensive Cancer Center/
University Hospitals Seidman Cancer Center and
Cleveland Clinic Taussig Cancer Institute
Cleveland, Ohio
UH Seidman Cancer Center
800.641.2422 • *uhhospitals.org/services/cancer-services*
CC Taussig Cancer Institute
866.223.8100 • *my.clevelandclinic.org/departments/cancer*
Case CCC
216.844.8797 • *case.edu/cancer*

City of Hope National Medical Center
Duarte, California
800.826.4673 • *cityofhope.org*

Dana-Farber/Brigham and Women's Cancer Center |
Mass General Cancer Center
Boston, Massachusetts
877.442.3324 • *youhaveus.org*
617.726.5130 • *massgeneral.org/cancer-center*

Duke Cancer Institute
Durham, North Carolina
888.275.3853 • *dukecancerinstitute.org*

Fox Chase Cancer Center
Philadelphia, Pennsylvania
888.369.2427 • *foxchase.org*

Fred & Pamela Buffett Cancer Center
Omaha, Nebraska
402.559.5600 • *unmc.edu/cancercenter*

Fred Hutchinson Cancer Center
Seattle, Washington
206.667.5000 • *fredhutch.org*

Huntsman Cancer Institute at the University of Utah
Salt Lake City, Utah
800.824.2073 • *healthcare.utah.edu/huntsmancancerinstitute*

Indiana University Melvin and Bren Simon
Comprehensive Cancer Center
Indianapolis, Indiana
888.600.4822 • *www.cancer.iu.edu*

Mayo Clinic Comprehensive Cancer Center
Phoenix/Scottsdale, Arizona
Jacksonville, Florida
Rochester, Minnesota
480.301.8000 • Arizona
904.953.0853 • Florida
507.538.3270 • Minnesota
mayoclinic.org/cancercenter

Memorial Sloan Kettering Cancer Center
New York, New York
800.525.2225 • *mskcc.org*

Moffitt Cancer Center
Tampa, Florida
888.663.3488 • *moffitt.org*

O'Neal Comprehensive Cancer Center at UAB
Birmingham, Alabama
800.822.0933 • *uab.edu/onealcancercenter*

Robert H. Lurie Comprehensive Cancer Center
of Northwestern University
Chicago, Illinois
866.587.4322 • *cancer.northwestern.edu*

Roswell Park Comprehensive Cancer Center
Buffalo, New York
877.275.7724 • *roswellpark.org*

Siteman Cancer Center at Barnes-Jewish Hospital
and Washington University School of Medicine
St. Louis, Missouri
800.600.3606 • *siteman.wustl.edu*

St. Jude Children's Research Hospital/
The University of Tennessee Health Science Center
Memphis, Tennessee
866.278.5833 • *stjude.org*
901.448.5500 • *uthsc.edu*

Stanford Cancer Institute
Stanford, California
877.668.7535 • *cancer.stanford.edu*

The Ohio State University Comprehensive Cancer Center -
James Cancer Hospital and Solove Research Institute
Columbus, Ohio
800.293.5066 • *cancer.osu.edu*

The Sidney Kimmel Comprehensive
Cancer Center at Johns Hopkins
Baltimore, Maryland
410.955.8964
www.hopkinskimmelcancercenter.org

The UChicago Medicine Comprehensive Cancer Center
Chicago, Illinois
773.702.1000 • *uchicagomedicine.org/cancer*

The University of Texas MD Anderson Cancer Center
Houston, Texas
844.269.5922 • *mdanderson.org*

UC Davis Comprehensive Cancer Center
Sacramento, California
916.734.5959 • 800.770.9261
health.ucdavis.edu/cancer

UC San Diego Moores Cancer Center
La Jolla, California
858.822.6100 • cancer.ucsd.edu

UCLA Jonsson Comprehensive Cancer Center
Los Angeles, California
310.825.5268 • uclahealth.org/cancer

UCSF Helen Diller Family
Comprehensive Cancer Center
San Francisco, California
800.689.8273 • cancer.ucsf.edu

University of Colorado Cancer Center
Aurora, Colorado
720.848.0300 • coloradocancercenter.org

University of Michigan Rogel Cancer Center
Ann Arbor, Michigan
800.865.1125 • rogelcancercenter.org

University of Wisconsin Carbone Cancer Center
Madison, Wisconsin
608.265.1700 • uwhealth.org/cancer

UT Southwestern Simmons
Comprehensive Cancer Center
Dallas, Texas
214.648.3111 • utsouthwestern.edu/simmons

Vanderbilt-Ingram Cancer Center
Nashville, Tennessee
877.936.8422 • vicc.org

Yale Cancer Center/Smilow Cancer Hospital
New Haven, Connecticut
855.4.SMILOW • yalecancercenter.org

We want your feedback!

Our goal is to provide helpful and easy-to-understand information on cancer.

Take our survey to let us know what we got right and what we could do better.

NCCN.org/patients/feedback

Index

Made in the USA
Monee, IL
16 May 2026

50326403R00038